# Della's Natural Diabetic Lifestyle

# Della's Natural Diabetic Lifestyle

## by

### Della M. Clare

Everlasting Publishing
Yakima, Washington
USA

*Della's Natural Diabetic Lifestyle*

*by*
*Della M. Clare*

Cover design by Jahla Brown

*ISBN: 0-9852739-3-3*

*ISBN-13: 978-0-9852739-3-4*

First Edition
Everlasting Publishing
P.O. Box 1061
Yakima, Washington 98907
USA

# Della's Natural Diabetic Lifestyle

# Table of Contents

*This book and the advice given herein is not intended to replace the program and instructions given you by your doctor to treat your diabetes, but to encourage you to follow the program and to suggest ways to adhere to it. I recommend that you follow your doctor's advice to the letter. Go to the classes your doctor suggests and follow the program.*

**If you want to live, follow the program.
If you don't, don't.**

# 1. INTRODUCTION

*Why I began this lifestyle*

Imagine my surprise when I discovered the assortment of my symptoms which I attributed to the aging process were not that at all. My hair was wispy and colorless, my tongue was coated so that food had no flavor, except for citrus drinks, and they became an odd necessity. I found myself making extra shopping trips in order to pick up another gallon or two of fruit juice in order to appease the thirstiness. But maybe, I said to myself, this is what happens when one gets older; the hair changes texture and food has a different flavor.

During the night, my body and my head were so hot. Could this be a reoccurrence of hot flashes? I found that thought to be reasonable. I would turn my pillow over several times, as I would awaken to the heated area, and search for cool spot. The same process would take place in trying to find a cooler location to move my feet and my body. The heat seemed to be coming from the inside of me, like a stove. Never had I heard anyone complain about hot flashes that fit the description, but this isn't a topic that is part of general conversations. So I dismissed any worrisome thoughts.

Although I didn't confide in my husband or to our son, since I presumed everything that was happening to me was normal, they noticed my behavior becoming more unusual throughout the weeks and months. One day, our son, who is a nurse, announced that he had made an appointment for me with our physician and I was to be there for tests. Of course, I complied, and shortly afterwards a call came that I had an exceptionally high glucose level, high blood pressure, high cholesterol; in fact, nothing in the chart was normal. I was shocked.

The doctor told me I had diabetes. One reason I was so stunned by this evaluation was because I have never been overweight. I am small, just five feet tall, and my weight has always been less than 100 pounds. I almost could not believe it was possible that I could be a diabetic... yet, this was what the doctor was telling me.

I wasn't familiar with anything concerning diabetes except that it was a disease. I was fortunate in that mine is the Type II. Immediately I was to begin taking the medication, which brought the glucose level down remarkably fast. My blood pressure and cholesterol were lowered within a few weeks.

The diabetes specialist urged me to attend classes also, and I began to learn everything I could about the disease. Within three months of medication, daily exercise, and careful attention to my food intake, I was able to be taken off the medication, and to control the diabetes naturally by following the suggested program.

As a result, I had a new growth of hair, with darker hair replacing the colorless. Food became so flavorful as my tongue lost the coating. My continual thirst was finally satisfied. All this was through the natural process, using no other medications or vitamins. Mother Nature is able to work wonders when we conclude that we must work with her instead of attempting to manipulate and govern or ignore her signals that manifest themselves into physical symptoms.

Therefore, for the diabetic it is imperative to modify or completely change the previous lifestyle. To conform to the program has life-saving rewards, of course, and in addition, I have made use of my personal observations that seem to be helpful, and ward off any depression that sometimes will arise after one receives the evaluation of the disease of diabetes.

The following information is from my personal experience and how I learned that diabetes can be managed for effective and pleasant results.

*Why this book was written*

- To supplement the program your doctor has given you

- To provide suggestions to the diabetic

- To encourage the reader

*Who can benefit from this book*

- Anyone recently diagnosed with diabetes

- People with a family history of diabetes

- People who are overweight

- People who want to change to a healthier lifestyle

## 2. MY PERSONAL TESTIMONY

When I first received the evaluation of having diabetes a few years ago, my doctor offered me some options. Since I was in the early stages and the disease had not progressed very far, he suggested I attempt to control it naturally by exercise and diet before he would start giving me insulin.

I was thrilled! I thought this must be the most fun disease to have, where all I needed to do to keep it under control was through healthy habits. I reviewed the list of foods (and amounts) I am allowed to eat, as well as the foods I needed to avoid. I made a decision right then and there that this was the prescription given to me by my doctor, and I needed to follow it faithfully. True, some of my favorite foods are on the list of foods I am not allowed to eat, but the list of allowed foods is so varied, with so many good foods! I found that by not buying foods with sugar in them, such as cookies, candy and ice cream, I had enough in my grocery budget to spend on a wider variety of fruits and vegetables. Since I am the primary cook and food shopper in our household, this aspect of my program would be easy for me to control.

I also made a decision about my exercise program. I thought, if I am too busy now to fit exercise into my lifestyle, when I can choose to follow this part of my prescription, the day may come when I will not be able to exercise at all - not because I'm too busy, but because I haven't taken care of my body and it will no longer function as it does now.

I began with my prescription of diet and exercise four years ago, and my diabetes is still under control, naturally, without the need for insulin. Each time I have gone in for my periodic check of my blood sugar levels, they have been well within the healthy range. I have followed the program my doctor suggested and made it my own healthy lifestyle.

Take the time to take care of yourself, your body and your health. Make the decision today to be healthy, and follow through on a daily basis. Each day choose to make the best decisions for the sake of your own health.

## 3. TAKING CARE OF YOURSELF BY TAKING CONTROL OF YOUR SITUATION

Today in this country we have an epidemic of diabetes. It is not contagious, but the lifestyle leading to becoming a diabetic can be, unless you are proactive about your health.

If your doctor told you to take pills or you will die, would you take the pills? If he or she told you to give yourself shots or you will die, would you do it? If your doctor told you to change your diet, eliminate certain foods and exercise daily or you will die, would you do it?

First and foremost: follow the instructions set forth by your doctor and diabetes specialist. Attend all of the classes. You will receive books and pamphlets on how to control your diabetes. Read them, study them, and reread them.

There are always a few people who resist the ideas. For example, one lady in our diabetes class, who has had the disease for many years rarely checked her glucose count with her home monitor. She said she hadn't checked it recently because once she cut herself and didn't want to waste the blood. She was at another class months later and complained that she felt sick all of the time. She was overweight and seemed to have lost no weight in that period of time.

Another lady complained because she just couldn't have a snack at her desk, plus her morning coffee was so important to her that she didn't want to take the medication and then wait to 30 minutes before she had any food or drink.

The instructors can only tell you and guide you; they can't do it for you. Your good health is up to you and you alone. That thought must be emphasized.

*Think of yourself first!*

That idea is contrary to our lifelong encouragement to 'share.' After your personal schedule has been established, plan everything else around that schedule. Appointments? Arrange them to coincide with your schedule; and that schedule is important. Meals, snacks and exercise need to be about the same time everyday. The reply is, "No, I can't come at that time, that is my walking time," (or snack time, etc.). "I'd love to have a piece of cake (pie, ice cream, cookies) but that is not in my menu."

Create your personal daily schedule, plan what time you will eat each meal and snack and what time you will exercise, and stick to it faithfully.

Put these things on your to-do list every day:

- Check your blood sugar.

- Check your blood pressure.

- Keep your feet covered and keep circulation to your feet. (I put lotion on my feet every morning, but not between toes, because they can get damp inside shoes.)

- Check your feet for tiny sores, especially if your feet have any numbness.

- Brush your teeth twice a day.

- Exercise. (Find something you really enjoy, enough to do it every day.)

- Eat your meals at specified times.

- Drink at least five glasses of water.

- If you smoke, quit now. (By the way, I smoked for years, but I did quit for good. You can quit smoking too, and it will be for your good.)

*Dental hygiene and diabetes*

I worked for a dentist for more than twenty years before I retired. I have learned that diabetics are at special risk for periodontal disease, an infection of the gums and bones that hold the teeth in place. Periodontal disease can lead to sore gums, painful chewing difficulties and eventually tooth loss. Dry mouth, frequently a symptom of undetected diabetes (which is why you often feel so thirsty), can cause soreness, mouth ulcers, infections, and tooth decay.

Smoking makes these problems worse. (Again, if you smoke, quit now!)

Controlling your blood glucose is key to controlling and preventing mouth problems. People with poor blood glucose control get gum disease more often and more severely than people whose diabetes is well-controlled. Daily brushing and flossing, regular dental check-ups and controlling your blood glucose are the best defense against the oral complications of diabetes.

## The importance of diet and nutrition to a diabetic

What you choose to eat: this is one area where you are in complete control, unless someone else puts food in your mouth at every meal. Are you the one planning meals for yourself and for your family? If you are that person, the meal-planner, good for you! You can help improve the health of your entire family by selecting healthy, nutritious foods for meals and snacks. Planning your shopping trips and your meals can be fun, and doing it faithfully will increase your chances of being successful in managing your diabetes. Failing to plan your meals will likely cause you to grow hungry and eat whatever is available. Grazing is not a good choice for anyone, and especially not for the person who has diabetes.

Even if you are not the one who shops and plans the meals for your family, you can give your family shopper a list of foods that you should be eating, as well as a no-no list of foods that you would prefer to not be brought into your house. You can also help with the family meal planning by suggesting to your family member meals that would be beneficial to your health as well as appetizing and nutritious for your whole family.

I came across three overweight ladies in the grocery store who were discussing counting calories. When they saw me one of them said to me, "You don't need to worry about that."

"Yes, I do, because I am trying to gain a few pounds and it's so hard," I said.

"What do you do?" another lady asked me.

I told them about my natural lifestyle of eating five small, regular meals each day and taking a one-hour walk every day, how I made a daily walking schedule and meal plan, and I stick to it.

"Well, then, stop doing that," the first lady said.

I started to laugh.

"When you get to be our age, you won't be able to walk like that," the third lady cautioned me.

"How old are you?" I asked.

"56. We are all 56," she answered.

"My son is your age!" I told them.

They gave me a second look and looked at me as if they didn't believe me.

Keep in mind: no sugar, salt or fat, and a whole new world of eating and planning meals will open for you. One person commented to me, "Those are all of the good things," in reference to the sugar, salt and fat. However, to eliminate those foods supplements does not suggest a future of bland meals. Spices and herbs are highly recommended for the diabetic, in that they stimulate the circulation of the physical processes.

To flavor your foods, add unsalted nuts, especially almonds, and seeds. No salt, of course, which means you are able to savor the flavors of the nuts and seeds you have selected.

Be a smart shopper and a smart eater. Take the time to read the labels. Make a conscious choice to think about what you are eating. Who is choosing your meals? Who is choosing your snacks? Who has control over what you eat? Do you have influence over your own or your family's food selections?

*A few words about portion control*

Measure your food. Learn to recognize how much is half a cup of rice, half a cup of cereal, two or three ounces of meat. Be aware of the amount of food you are eating.

Did you know you can trick yourself into eating smaller amounts by using a smaller plate? Try it. Fill a smaller plate than you usually use and after you eat, you will feel as full as when you use a larger plate. We are so conditioned to eat everything on our plates, we will be as satisfied by eating a smaller plate full of food as we are when we eat a larger plate full of food.

Have you noticed how portions served by restaurants are so much larger than they were in the past? When ordering in a restaurant, ask for a box and then take home half of your meal. And just because they offer you free refills on your drinks, you don't need to take them.

*Why is it so difficult to stop eating sugar?*

We are constantly being flooded with advertisements for sugar. You can't turn on the TV or look on the Internet or read any kind of magazine without seeing a multitude of ads for products that contain sugar. The media is bombarding us with the idea that if we don't drink this sugary drink or eat this sugary food, nobody will like us. Their message to us: if you fill yourself full of sugar every day by eating and drinking these specific sugary items, you will be popular and asked to partake in all kinds of fun and wonderful activities. The truth is (and remember, I worked for a dentist for many years) that if you drink sugary drinks every day, you will be at risk of losing your teeth. You can also easily add pounds that sneak up on you along with the added sugar. How popular will you be when that happens?

So many food items contain sugar, besides the obvious: candy, cookies, cakes, ice cream, donuts, pastries, pies, pop. Even 'healthy' foods contain sugar (read the labels, look for sugar, corn syrup, fructose, sucrose): yogurt, granola bars, crackers, peanut butter (buy peanut butter which contains only peanuts, peanut oil and salt), frozen fruits, canned vegetables,and breads. Many low-fat foods contain sugar: low fat does not mean low sugar. Again, check the ingredients of all your food to be sure the manufacturers did not sneak in sugar by some other name.

Beware: you may be eating much more sugar than you think you are eating, without knowing it, because sugar has a multitude of names, as it is disguised inside other foods. Can you believe sugar has more than fifty different names? As you check the ingredients on packages, notice how sugar is called by so many names, to keep you guessing at how much total sugar the product actually contains.

Here are some of the most common (or not) names of sugar:
- Agave nectar
- Barley malt
- Buttered syrup
- Cane juice
- Cane sugar
- Caramel
- Carob syrup
- Corn syrup
- Dextran

- Dextrose
- Diastatic malt
- Florida crystals
- Fructose
- Galactose
- Glucose
- Golden syrup
- High-fructose corn syrup
- Honey
- Lactose
- Maltodextrine
- Maltose
- Maple syrup
- Molasses
- Raw sugar
- Rice syrup
- Sucrose
- Turbinado sugar

Watch for these names when you are reading the ingredient list on packages, and you will begin to notice: sugar by any other name is still sugar.

The best way to cut sugar out of your menu completely is to eat natural foods (fruits, vegetables, meats and breads) and prepare your own meals so you know exactly what goes into them.  When you choose to eat processed and packaged food and fast food, you can't accurately measure the amount of sugar you are eating. However, you can be sure when you eat processed, packaged and fast foods, you are eating more sugar than you think you are eating.

A few tips to help you cut sugar out of your diet.
- Eliminate sugary drinks. This includes soda pop, sugary waters and sweetened coffee and tea drinks.

- Stop eating sugary snacks. Candy, cookies, cake, ice cream muffins (even the ones that sound 'healthy,' like banana nut and wheat bran are secretly loaded with sugar), granola bars (sugar has been sneaked in to them, too) and donuts. (My mother taught me that donuts were triple threats to our health: deep-fried sugary white flour dipped in sugar.)

- Reduce sugars found in white flour products, such as bread, crackers, white rice and pasta. Substitute whole-wheat for white flour breads and pasta, brown rice for white rice, and again, I urge you to check those ingredients.

Currently, there is a debate regarding whether or not sugar is addictive. I can tell you from personal experience, to me, I was addicted to it. When I eat sugar first thing in the morning, perhaps a donut or sugary cereal, I crave sugar all day long. After I have eaten something with high sugar content, I want to eat more sugar. I find myself searching for something sweet to eat. The sweet-loving portion of my tongue has been activated and it wants more and more. The day after I eat too much sugar, when I determine that I am not going to eat anything that contains sugar, I begin to get a headache. I feel sluggish and my digestion slows to a crawl. These are my sugar withdrawal symptoms. Yes, I literally have withdrawal symptoms when I stop eating sugar.

I challenge you to stop eating sugar, stop completely. Will you make excuses as to why you can't stop eating sugar? Will you tell me that you can stop eating sugar any time you want, but at this time, you just don't want to stop? You decide for yourself whether or not you think it is addictive.

*Some of the results I experienced when I stopped eating sugar*

My hair had begun to turn gray when I was in my 70s, before I had received the evaluation of being a diabetic. I accepted this as a part of the aging process. A few weeks after I stopped eating sugar, I went to get my hair cut. My hairdresser, the only person who closely examines my hair, was amazed. He remarked, "Your hair is growing back brown!" He plucked out a strand and showed it to me, and sure enough, the new growth was back to my original hair color! About a month later, I could see in the mirror that the gray of my hair was disappearing and my hair was turning all brown again. I began to look younger without any hair dye or any type of artificial hair treatment.

My tongue had been coated, and I thought it was another symptom of the aging process. After I stopped eating sugar, my tongue is clear and I am able to taste flavors better than ever!

The day after I stopped eating sugar, I immediately had more energy. I was not getting tired, as I had been previously (also, I had attributed *that* to old age) and I had all the energy I needed to do all the things I wanted to do.

The craving I had had for sugar and sweets stopped. I was like a recovered addict, finally able to select healthy foods over sweets. I no longer needed to hunt down the nearest piece of chocolate or gumdrop in order to feel satisfied. Instead, I began to crave fruits and I wanted to eat them every day.

Within a couple of days after I stopped eating sugar, the night sweats stopped! I was so happy when I was finally able to sleep the entire night in cool comfort. I felt like a new person every morning, cool and refreshed.

My memory improved! Those foggy thoughts, or not remembering why I came into this room (or why I went downstairs or upstairs) were no longer a part of my mental state. I was able to remember things so much better, which helped me feel like I was getting younger instead of getting older.

Another tip: Do not eat sugar replacements. They are chemicals your body does not need and these chemicals are, in fact, harmful to your body. When you see any of these items listed as an ingredient, do not buy or eat the food that contains it: aspartame, sucralose, neotame, acesulfame potassium (Ace-K), saccharin, and advantame.

## Water: the Key to Life

Drinking water is important to the diabetic. You should drink at least five 8-ounce glasses of water each day to stay hydrated, which helps control your blood sugar. More than five glasses of water per day is even better for you. Why does staying hydrated help control blood sugar? Being too dry tells your kidneys to hold onto water and tells the liver to release stored blood sugar. It also raises your blood pressure. Extra sugar should be passed out of the body in urine, but if there is not much water in your system, the kidneys don't make urine.

Not drinking water can lead to over-eating and weight gain. In many Americans, the thirst mechanism is so unrecognizable that it is often mistaken for hunger. Dehydration also slows down the body's metabolism and digestive system and is a major cause of fatigue.

What if you drink plenty of coffee or tea or juice or milk or diet pop? Do you still need to drink five glasses of water each day? Yes, because every other drink besides water requires your body to process it.

Plain water is what your body needs, not any other type of liquid. You can drink these other fluids in moderation, but they do not count toward your daily water allotment.

My suggestion regarding diet pop (soda): don't drink it. For one thing, the artificial sweeteners trigger the craving for sweets; and, more importantly, have you looked at the ingredients? Do you know what chemicals diet pop contains? Can you even pronounce the names of those chemicals? I advise you to not eat or drink anything if you don't know what it is or what it contains.

# 4. SHOPPING LISTS (FOOD TO ALWAYS HAVE AT HOME)

*Vegetables*
- Peppers and onions – to add to egg sandwiches, wraps, breakfast burritos, omelets, quick stir-fry dishes
- Fresh tomatoes – these also go well with sandwiches and wraps, or cut them up and use in salads and cottage cheese
- Fresh baby carrots, cherry tomatoes, snap peas and precut vegetables are quick to snack and pack. Also keep some basic salad ingredients like spinach and mixed greens, a cucumber and zucchini
- Broccoli, cauliflower, bell peppers and celery; chop them up when you get home to use throughout the week
- Frozen vegetables – keep a few of your favorites in the freezer
- Canned vegetables: reduced-sodium canned tomatoes, artichoke hearts, roasted red peppers, olives
- Canned or bottled vegetable juice (be sure vegetables are the only ingredients)

*Whole grains*

- Quick oats (can be ready in less than 2 minutes)

- 100% whole-wheat bread or whole-wheat English muffins

- Unsweetened whole grain or bran cereal

- 100% whole-wheat bread, pitas, or wraps – consider a low-carb version

- Quinoa, barley, brown rice

*Eggs & dairy*

- Eggs or egg substitute

- Skim or 1% milk – soy milk or almond milk are also good options, especially for those with a lactose intolerance or dairy sensitivity

- Light or non-fat yogurt (regular or Greek) – plain is best, since it contains less sugar than flavored varieties

- Cottage cheese – low-fat or non-fat

- Parmesan cheese, to sprinkle on salads and vegetables

*Fruit*

- Fresh fruit – apples, bananas, oranges, tangerines, pears, mangoes, nectarines, peaches, cherries and berries in season

- Frozen fruit – blueberries, raspberries, strawberries, blackberries, cherries, mangoes and peaches to use in smoothies or to mix with yogurt

- Packaged fruit – individual-size cups of mandarin oranges, pineapple, peaches or fruit cocktail (in juice or water, not syrup)
- Dried fruit – raisins and dried cranberries are great in oatmeal or mixed with nuts
- Fresh berries and grapes, easy to wash and serve in a bowl
- Lemons and limes – juice from these citrus fruits makes a great flavoring for vegetables, fish or chicken
- Whole fruit jams and jellies (no sugar or artificial sweetener added)

*Protein foods*
- Canned tuna
- Reduced-sodium canned beans – pinto, black, kidney, red, navy, garbanzo, small white beans, lentils
- Reduced-sodium lean deli meat – roasted turkey, chicken or roast beef
- Eggs – hard boil ahead of time to eat alone or in salads, or use in quick scrambles
- Unsalted nuts or nut mix
- Rotisserie chicken – use it throughout the week in salads, pastas, sandwiches or tacos
- Frozen chicken or fish filets (not breaded)
- Extra lean ground beef

*Starchy foods*
- Whole-grain pasta, whole-wheat cous cous

- Brown rice, whole-wheat or corn tortillas
- Potatoes, sweet potatoes

*Nuts (add to salads and other vegetable dishes)*
- Unsalted nuts – dry roasted walnuts, pecans, almonds, peanuts or mixed nuts
- Pistachios and peanuts in the shell require to slow down to eat them (choose unsalted, roasted or unroasted)
- Natural peanut butter and/or almond butter – nut butters will keep you feeling full and satisfy your craving for something smooth

*Additional items to always have on hand*
- Olive oil
- Balsamic vinegar
- Various spices and dried herbs
- Hot sauce
- Hummus
- Mustard
- Sea salt and pepper
- Minced garlic (jarred)
- Salsa
- Lime and/or lemon juice
- Light salad dressing (check the ingredient list on dressings – better yet, make your own dressing; see recipes)

# 5. SUGGESTED MEAL PLANS AND RECIPES

I love bread. I love it fresh. I love it toasted. I love it with butter. I love it with jam. I could eat bread all day long. But I don't. I make a plan for the week and do my grocery shopping once a week, according to that plan. (I don't want to spend my time going to the store every day to try to find something for dinner.) Following a plan will help us keep our blood sugar balanced, and keep us alive and healthy.

One day I was at the store, selecting fruits and vegetables for the week and a lady started a conversation with me. The subject came up that we both were following the diabetic diet.

"Sometimes I cheat," she confided to me.

"Who are you cheating?" I asked her.

Her mouth dropped open and she gave me the strangest look as she seemed consider her reply. She walked away from me without saying anything more.

Often times we don't know what to eat. We just look for something appealing, something handy.

This is the reason we need to make a plan, a specific meal plan, for every meal of every day.

For the diabetic, five or six small meals each day can be better than two or three large meals. Smaller meals spread throughout the day help keep your blood sugar at a consistent level. When you eat only two or three large meals per day, you run the risk of letting your blood sugar level drop too low if the meals are too far apart, or, if you eat a large meal, and especially if you add dessert, your blood sugar level can easily creep up or spike to dangerously high levels.

You can have fun with your meal planning! You know what you like to eat, and you can best select foods that are most nutritious and tasty to you. It is very important for the diabetic to choose to eat the healthiest food possible and to have regular meal times. When you select healthy foods that you enjoy, you will be more likely to stick to your meal plan, and you will, in fact, look forward to each meal and your tummy will be ready at the specific time.

*Quick and healthy breakfast ideas*

When I start my day with a healthy meal, I want to keep it up all day long. We have so many options!

Scrambled egg: Whisk together an egg with a tablespoon of milk, some garlic power and black pepper. After cooking in the microwave for about one minute, when the egg is done, top with a tablespoon of salsa and a tablespoon of low-fat cheese.

Breakfast burrito: Scramble an egg and microwave for 30-60 seconds. When the egg is done, wrap it in a whole-wheat tortilla with some sliced bell peppers and tomatoes. Top with a dash of hot sauce, wrap in a paper towel, waxed paper or foil and bring with you. (Or eat it at home.)

Cold cereal: Prepare a small bowl of whole grain or bran cereal with 1/2 cup of non-fat milk or almond milk. Top with fresh berries, dried fruit or nuts.

Smoothie: Use 1/2 cup of non-fat plain Greek yogurt, 2 tablespoons low-fat milk, soy milk or almond milk and 1/2 cup of fresh or frozen fruit. Blend it all together and bring it with you on the go. You could also add a tablespoon of peanut butter, some ground flax or a sprinkle of cinnamon.

Yogurt parfait: In a dish, layer 1/2 cup plain Greek non-fat yogurt, 1/2 cup berries and some chopped pecans or a tablespoon of unsweetened granola.

Peanut butter and toast: Toast a slice of 100% whole-wheat bread or whole-wheat English muffin. Top with 1-2 tablespoons of natural peanut butter or almond butter.

Cottage cheese and peaches: Half a cup of cottage cheese and half a cup canned peaches. If you don't like peaches, use cherries or pineapple, raspberries, blueberries or even diced tomatoes. Add a small handful of nuts on the side if desired.

Microwave oats: Mix 1/4 cup of quick oats with 1/2 cup water or non-fat milk and cook in the microwave for about one minute or until oats are cooked. Stir in some cinnamon and a small handful of dry roasted nuts. Add an apple on the side or mix in a tablespoon of dried fruit if desired. Or add diced apple with cinnamon to your oatmeal, especially good together.

Make-ahead-overnight-no-cook-oatmeal: Ratio should be about 1 part oats + 2 parts milk + 1/4 part seeds. Combine milk (or almond milk or soy milk), oats, Chia seeds (or flax seeds, pumpkin seeds or unsalted sunflower seeds), and cinnamon in a 1/2-pint jar with a lid; cover and shake until combined. Remove lid and fold in cherries or berries. Cover jar with lid. Refrigerate overnight. If berries are frozen, thaw in separate container in refrigerator and add to oatmeal in the morning.

Try these healthier choices when fast food is your only option in the morning.

Small latte made with skim milk (or almond milk) and a package of nuts and/or a small piece of fruit to go with it.

Oatmeal with fresh or dried fruit and nuts.

Small fruit-yogurt parfait with a cup of coffee.

For a hot breakfast, try an egg and cheese breakfast sandwich or wrap. Add extra vegetables, if possible, and skip the fatty meats (bacon and sausage).

## Lunch: a variety of suggestions

Sandwich alternatives: Use two pieces of thin sandwich bread or a whole-wheat tortilla wrap with two ounces low-sodium lean turkey, spinach, bell pepper and mustard. Add some carrot sticks and light ranch dressing or guacamole on the side.

Tuna salad: Use canned tuna, light mayonnaise or plain Greek yogurt, diced celery, lemon juice and freshly ground pepper. Serve on greens with an apple and peanut butter on the side.

Lettuce wrap: Wrap low-fat meat or tuna salad in lettuce instead of bread.

Grain salad: Mix together some cooked quinoa, white beans, chopped bell pepper, carrots and broccoli. Toss with a bit of olive oil, lemon juice, salt and pepper. Add a tangerine or nectarine or some grapes on the side and a small handful of almonds.

Leftover chili or vegetable soup: Top with fresh tomatoes and non-fat plain yogurt instead of sour cream.

Whole-wheat wrap: Fill a whole-wheat tortilla wrap with leftover chicken, hummus, sun-dried tomatoes, feta cheese and greens. Add a side of fruit.

Hard-boiled egg, fruit, string cheese and 5 whole-wheat crackers. You could also add some carrots, celery sticks and peanut butter.

Salad with romaine lettuce or spinach and any other non-starchy vegetables that you like. Top with cottage cheese, chopped nuts and a tablespoon of light dressing.

Mediterranean turkey wrap: Spread 2 tablespoons hummus on whole-wheat wrap. Top with 3 ounces turkey, 1/4 cup cucumber, 1/4 cup tomatoes, 1 tablespoon feta cheese and 1 diced olive. Fold wrap to close.

Greek salad: Dice half a cucumber, half a green bell pepper, one tomato, one slice of red onion, five large olives (black or Kalamata) and one tablespoon feta cheese.

## Lunch suggestions at restaurants

Choose grilled meat, fish, and poultry over fried.

Try a vegetarian option, such as a grilled vegetable wrap with fresh vegetables and hummus.

Salad with the dressing on the side. (Ask for less cheese and hold the fried onions and meats.)

Order the smallest sandwich, not the double burger or large sandwich. Select the 6-inch sub instead of the foot-long sub sandwich.

Ask if whole-wheat is an option for sandwich bread, wraps, or pitas.

Choose fresh vegetables, fresh fruit or low-fat yogurt as side dishes instead of fries or onion rings.

Ask for a broth-based vegetable or bean soup instead of creamy soup.

## Nutritious Dinner Ideas

When I plan dinners for the week, my method is simple: chicken, chicken, pork, chicken, chicken, beef. I am not fond of turkey and I don't care for fish, but you can add those into your dinner planning, if you like them. You may also choose vegetarian meals for your dinner plan, but I like to stick to my rotation of chicken, pork and beef. Once a week I serve leftovers for dinner, to complete the seven days.

My favorite soup recipe is not only simple, but simply delicious. Begin with some water in a container and add every spice in your cupboard, garlic, ginger, dill weed, pepper, oregano, basil, sage, chili, vinegar as examples, and everything else that appeals to you. Then add navy beans or lentils or barley or noodles or a combination. These vegetables add flavor and are nutritious also: onions, celery, cabbage, red and green peppers. (Raw vegetables are the best, of course, but in the soup they add color in addition to the flavors.) Simmer the mixture with pieces of chicken or with beef (low fat hamburger, for example, that has been browned) for two or three hours, and enjoy your 'original' recipe.

Mashed potatoes can be more appetizing with the addition of a few spices, since gravy is not on our list of recommended foods. Add some garlic, low fat sour cream, pepper, a wee bit of basil, plus a small amount of low fat milk. Who needs the gravy?

A delicious alternative to mashed potatoes is mashed cauliflower. Cut the head of cauliflower into small pieces and boil or steam until it becomes soft. Then smash it with a potato masher and add a little bit of butter, garlic and pepper. (I suggest that you do not use the spice called 'garlic pepper' because it is made up of mostly salt. Check the ingredients of everything you eat.)

For fruit or fruit salads, sprinkle with cinnamon. It not only enhances the flavor of the fruit, but cinnamon lowers the glucose level. I like to add a spoonful of plain yogurt to my fruit salad. Nutmeg, cloves and any other spice that appeals to the diabetic also is delectable to the non-diabetic. Thus the meals and the snacks need not seem restrictive, just different and more interesting. For example, a fresh apple with a bit of cinnamon tastes like apple pie or applesauce. The reward? No sugar to jeopardize the blood sugar count. (Cinnamon is good also with peaches and bananas, too.)

Here is a very quick dish; this one can be a side dish or a main dish:
- Can of beans (black beans, pinto beans, kidney beans or small white beans)
- Can of no-salt diced tomatoes (use Italian or Mexican-spiced versions for variety)
- Can of corn

Rinse and drain beans and corn before adding to pot. Stir ingredients as you gently heat. Or heat in the microwave.

Vegetarian chili: Chop one medium onion, one green bell pepper, one zucchini, one sweet potato and four carrots and add to pot with one tablespoon of canola oil. Cook for about 5 minutes, stirring regularly. Add two cloves of minced garlic and one tablespoon of chili powder (use mild, medium or hot, according to your taste). Add one can of kidney or pinto beans (rinsed and drained), one can of black beans (rinsed and drained), one can of tomato sauce and one can of no-salt diced tomatoes. Bring to a boil, then reduce heat and simmer for about half an hour.

Roasted whole chicken is very easy to make. Just put the whole chicken in a roaster, add lemon and herbs or a small amount of butter, garlic and pepper and cook in the oven at 350 degrees until it's done. Serve with vegetables and roasted garlic potatoes (See recipe below).

A great side dish I love to make is roasted garlic potatoes. Wash (no need to peel! Potato peelings are good for you) and then cut potatoes into large, bite-size chunks, spray with olive oil and toss with garlic powder, sea salt and black pepper in a bowl, then bake on a cookie sheet in the oven for about 30 minutes or until done.

Another chicken dish that is delicious: Cut up one chicken and boil for five minutes. Add a mixture of spices, such as dried onion, black pepper, parsley, basil, cayenne pepper, oregano, sage, garlic and turmeric, (which will turn the rice a beautiful yellow tint). Add one diced onion, three diced potatoes and one head of cut-up cauliflower to the boiling water, let boil for a few more minutes. Add one cup of brown rice and let it simmer for about 45 minutes or until the rice is done. Served topped with sautéed slivered almonds for a delight you will truly enjoy.

If you love fried chicken, try baking it instead, first coat the pieces with a beaten egg, then roll them in corn meal or crushed crackers and then bake in the oven. You will eliminate the fat and calories from the frying oil and you will love it as much as you love it fried.

Meatloaf: Add to your ground beef two grated carrots, one egg, 1/4 cup bulgur, half a cup of oatmeal and half a cup of low-sodium V-8 juice. Bake over sliced potatoes for a real treat.

Easy beef stew: I'm sure you have your favorite recipe, but I love to make it the traditional way with beef chunks, potatoes, carrots and onions. Add two tablespoons of whole-wheat flour to thicken the broth. The longer you cook it, the better it tastes, as the flavors blend together.

Pork chops with chicken soup (recipe from my mother): Spread mustard on pork chops (both sides), dip in whole-wheat flour and fry lightly on both sides. Transfer to baking pan or roaster and add one can of chicken noodle soup, half a cup of rice and one cup of water. Bake at 350 for one hour. (You may add more mustard to the mixture for a more tangy taste.)

Clam chowder (recipe from my mother): Cook

two strips of bacon and one small onion (diced). Transfer to pot with peeled, diced potatoes, and one cup of water. Bring to boil and boil five minutes. Reduce heat, add one can of minced clams and half a cup of cream. (Use milk or low-fat milk for a lower fat option.)

Stir-fry options: You can use any kind of meat to make a quick and easy, yet healthy, stir fry dinner. Leftover cooked chicken, pork or beef, or even frozen shrimp cooked with a small amount of canola or olive oil and a bag of frozen vegetables will have dinner on your table in just a few minutes. Serve over brown rice or whole-wheat noodles.

Chicken tacos: Use leftover chicken and fill a corn or whole-wheat tortilla with chopped or shredded chicken, tomatoes, lettuce, fresh cilantro and black beans. Top it with a spoonful of salsa and/ or non-fat plain Greek yogurt.

Chicken enchilada casserole: Layer whole-wheat or corn tortillas with diced chicken, diced onions, canned corn (rinsed and drained), just a little cheddar cheese and cover each layer with enchilada sauce. Make two to four layers high, depending on the depth of your baking dish. Top with a sprinkle of cheese. Bake in the oven for 45 minutes if chicken is already cooked, one hour if the chicken is not cooked. This is especially good with refried beans and Spanish rice on the side.

Salad as your dinner entrée: Chop up your favorite non-starchy vegetables and serve over a bed of greens. Add some rotisserie chicken breast and cottage cheese or another reduced-fat cheese. Have your salad with a side of whole-wheat bread or some fresh fruit.

Scrambled eggs with spinach for dinner: Top with diced peppers (red, yellow, orange or green) and green onions. Eat with a slice of whole-wheat toast.

Veggie flatbread: Sauté frozen or fresh vegetables and pile them onto a whole-wheat pizza crust (or a whole-wheat pita) and top with reduced-fat mozzarella cheese and tomato slices; or top with spinach, olives and feta cheese. Bake in the oven until the cheese melts.

This one is not my favorite, but here is a fish suggestion: Defrost frozen fish filets in the refrigerator the night before you plan to cook them. Brush fish lightly with olive oil and season with freshly ground pepper and other dried herbs. Bake the fish in the oven until done and serve with half a cup of brown rice and steamed green beans.

Do you have a bread maker? For heaven's sake, then make your own whole-grain bread! You will have control over the exact ingredients and it will be healthier than store-bought, as well as delicious.

*Healthy salad dressing you can make*
- Ranch dip/dressing: Use plain yogurt. Stir in spices, including basil, parsley, sage, garlic powder, onion powder, black pepper and sea salt.

- Tahini dressing: Blend together tahini, lemon juice, garlic, sea salt and water. Adjust amounts of ingredients to your liking (more or less lemon, more or less garlic).

- Try sprinkling Balsamic vinegar or lemon juice on your salad as a dressing.

*Snack suggestions*
- Half an apple and 8-10 unsalted almonds.

- Slice of whole-wheat toast, spread with unsweetened applesauce and cinnamon (One of my favorites, almost like a little slice of apple pie).

- Celery with peanut butter.

- Nutty snack mix: almonds, peanuts, sunflower seeds, walnuts, raisins.

- Roasted pumpkin seeds.

- Roasted garbanzo beans.

- 1/3 cup hummus with 1/2 cup mixed vegetable sticks.

- 1/2 cup yogurt with 2 tablespoons of granola.

- Pistachio nuts – just a handful.

- Tuna on 6 whole grain crackers.

- Angel eggs: Hard boil and half eggs and remove yokes. Blend yokes with avocado and spoon into egg white halves.

# 6. EXERCISE AND THE DIABETIC

*Why is exercise so important to the diabetic?*

Regular physical activity is a key part of managing diabetes, along with proper meal planning, taking medications as prescribed, and stress management. Exercising consistently can lower the blood glucose level, the main sugar found in the blood and the body's main source of energy. As a matter of fact, exercising can be your super weapon to control, treat, or even cure your diabetes. You will feel the effects of exercise almost instantly, as more oxygen begins to travel through your blood and to all the cells of your body as you begin to lower your insulin resistance. Believe me, a brisk walk or jog or bike ride will improve your entire being, from your state of mind to your spiritual being to your physical body, and you will feel it.

Make your exercise fun. Engage in activities that appeal to you. My husband and my son love to ski, ride their bikes, play volleyball and golf, and my niece loves to ice skate and roller skate. The great thing about exercising is that you can choose to do what you enjoy. That is the key, because if you don't enjoy it, you won't continue to do it on a regular basis. You will be more likely to do what you like to do.

I don't care for the physical pain associated with strenuous workouts, but I do enjoy the walking. That is the time when I meditate and contemplate the universal issues and consequently I have arrived at some interesting solutions and understanding in reference to Universal Harmony and the Law of Divine Power, what it is and how it works. In addition to these weighty subjects, my daily walks have added a lighter viewpoint. I have met and become acquainted with several neighbors who have lived in the area for many years, as we have; young parents, too, out with babies in strollers. Some of the children who were tiny when I first met them are old enough now to recognize me. It warms my heart to spend a few minutes talking and enjoying their smiling responses.

And I have to mention the dogs along my route. I am well acquainted with a certain few. One man stopped his car in the bicycle lane, opened his window and said, "Missy, look who's here." Missy looked around and came to the window and gave me a generously wet greeting. We get along just fine.

Two little poodles are often on a walk at the same time I am, and they get so excited when they see me down the block. They pull at their leashes until the owner has to let go, so they can run to meet me. They're so cute and so happy, which, in turn, makes me happy. Their owner beams.

Then there is the Springer Spaniel name Reggie that is a funny, funny dog. The house where he lives is fenced, so he runs as hard as he can to the gate and barks so viciously at me as I am walking by his house. One day his owner brought him outside the gate to meet me, and lo and behold, he was quiet and pleasant. He licked my hand and then gazed off to something else. Sometimes though, he is not in the mood for barking up a storm, so he will trot to the gate, bark a few barks, and go back. One very hot day, he was sitting in the shade, and when I called "Reggie," he looked up, replied, "Arf!" and remained in the shade. Another day he wasn't in the mood at all, so when I called, he looked up, took a few steps, made a small circle and hid behind some shrubs. I could see him peeking at me. I had to laugh aloud.

These humorous events are exceptionally beneficial to the physical system, in that every time a pleasant sensation occurs, as in a smile or a laugh, the body reacts in a positive way. Diabetics need to be aware of the importance of maintaining a happy attitude. Singing, too, is helpful. If nothing seems to be especially cheerful, find something! There is humor all around us.

What began a few years as a one-hour daily walk when I first started this journey has now extended to a two-hour daily walk, because I have met so many people on my route and I love to talk to them every day. What surprises will you encounter on your journey?

## Adding steps to your life

Be mindful of the steps you take every day, and make a conscious effort to increase the amount. If you have stairs in your house, go up and down several times daily. We have a basement in our house, and every day I find reasons to go downstairs and do something. When you are going up a stairway, don't just drag your feet up to the next step, but make it a habit to spring yourself up the stairs. This is a great way to get exercise in your own home.

One time a friend urged me to use a step-counter, and I was curious to see how much I walk during the day. I was not surprised to learn that I walk three miles during my outside walk, but I was astonished to discover that I walk nearly three miles inside my house every day!

When you go to the store, don't look for the parking space nearest the door. Park as far as possible from the door and walk quickly across the parking lot. Save the parking spaces near the door for those who can't walk, and be thankful that you can. When my sister comes to visit me, she gets a little upset with me when we go shopping at the mall because I park at the outer edge of the parking lot, then I make her walk with me once around the outside of the mall before we go inside and start our shopping.

# 7. PRAYER AND STRESS RELIEF / RELAXATION

Another factor to be taken into consideration when dealing with any chronic disease is to keep in touch with your inner being. As we have heard, "as within, same without," or, to quote from Proverbs, "For as a man thinketh in his heart, so is he." Think positive thoughts about yourself and envision your body healing itself as you follow this natural lifestyle. Encourage yourself to take the best care of yourself that you possibly can. After all, the Bible tells us to "Love your neighbor as yourself." It does not say to love your neighbor more than you love yourself; it says to love yourself too. This means to pay attention to your own personal care, especially in the case of the diabetic. A balance is needed between nutrition, exercise, work, play and stress relief or relaxation.

The diabetic must take time daily, or even better, several times each day, to relax so you can pray and meditate. We are all so busy these days. Take a break from whatever you have been doing, right now. Close your eyes and take a long, slow, deep breath, hold it for three seconds, and then slowly exhale. This will take about nine seconds (three seconds to inhale, three seconds to hold it, three seconds to release) and I don't believe anyone in this world does not have nine seconds to breathe and be refreshed. You can even spend a few extra seconds smiling, as your body enjoys the gift of relief you just gave to yourself.

Set aside a little time every day for reading something inspirational. Pick out a devotional book or a poetry book or even a humorous magazine, or read a few verses from the Bible. Even reading just for a few minutes each day can do wonders for improving your state of mind.

Prayer, meditation, and contemplation are beneficial in achieving a balance of the mind and body, which is to say they are one and the same. When we recognize the interdependence of the functions of the mind and body, the results are remarkable when the physical, mental and spiritual faculties are coordinated. Thus a corresponding response must follow the supplication in the form of thank You, thank You, thank You, to our God who makes all things possible.

# 8. SO WHAT ARE YOU GOING TO DO ABOUT IT?

I personally have received many benefits by following this natural lifestyle approach to living with diabetes. Now I am in my late 70s and I feel as healthy – or healthier – than I ever have felt in my life. I am sleeping well at night, I feel energized during the day, and I enjoy the routine and familiarity of having a plan in place, a daily guide to follow in terms of exercise, meal planning and eating, drinking water, my prayer and meditation time (I still stand on my head every day), shopping, and sleeping.

I am retired, and with my schedule I still have plenty of time left for my husband, my sons (I have two), my grandchildren (six girls and two boys), my great-grandchildren (five great-grandsons and one great granddaughter), and my other family members (my sister, my nieces and nephews and my cousins), my cats (three inside cats and the many I care for in our yard), and for my reading, which is one of my favorite activities. I am enjoying life to its fullest and my body is thanking me every day for taking care of it.

I am not saying that everyone will enjoy these same benefits, but I am telling you that I do. I don't have to say I am too tired to exercise, or too sore to exercise, or too busy to make the right choices regarding what I eat. I make a plan and I stick to it. This is my lifestyle and I am embracing it. I see people nearly every day who are half my age, but not even half as healthy as I am, and it is all because of what they choose to do and choose to not do.

These complications of advanced diabetes you can avoid by following your program (the program given to you by your doctor and your diabetes classes):
- Kidney damage
- Nerve damage
- Heart damage
- Kidney failure
- Loss of sensation (feeling in extremities)
- Loss of sense of taste and smell
- Blindness
- Amputations

You do not have to suffer any of these consequences. You can turn your sickness, your tiredness into your healthy self. You can do it, just like I did, by taking control of your habits. However, I must repeat, do not think you can simply follow the exact routine that I follow. You need to follow the instructions given to you by your doctor and follow the plan that you learn in your classes about caring for yourself and your diabetes.

A good attitude is very important. Be positive. You can do it. Do you want to make a difference in your own life? You are the only one who can make the choices to make that difference. Don't put the blame on anyone else if you are not eating the right foods, you are not exercising and you are still smoking. (Once again, if you smoke, stop now!) Making healthy choices on a daily basis will positively impact your life daily. You will see a difference the first day you choose a natural, healthy lifestyle. Educating yourself about the disease and coming to the realization that making your own healthy choices each day is the best way you can get healthy.

*Thank you to my niece, Dana Lynn Pride, for your assistance with getting this information from my pen and paper to others who may need it.*

*Love, Yaya*

www.ingramcontent.com/pod-product-compliance
Lightning Source LLC
Chambersburg PA
CBHW060642280326
41933CB00012B/2125